Get Rid Of Fat

Lose Love Handles

Table of Contents

These are some of my other books below, and my website is
www.LosingBellyFatMission.com :

https://www.amazon.com/dp/B06XB4WHZX
http://www.amazon.com/dp/B06X9LXBB8
http://www.amazon.com/dp/B06WLK7497
http://www.amazon.com/dp/B06W54JKQN
http://www.amazon.com/dp/B06X6DJ9K3
http://www.amazon.com/dp/B06WGNJ9N3
http://www.amazon.com/dp/B06W549TBD
http://www.amazon.com/dp/B06VTF5DQJ
http://www.amazon.com/dp/B06WRPSBKK
http://www.amazon.com/dp/B06WD194JR
http://www.amazon.com/dp/B06WCZTK7Y
http://www.amazon.com/dp/B06X3QN1HT
http://www.amazon.com/dp/B01N19WBF2
http://www.amazon.com/dp/B01N2AVECA
http://www.amazon.com/dp/B01N4VZIAV
http://www.amazon.com/dp/B00QJJFS1C
http://www.amazon.com/dp/B01EMNO2MW
http://www.amazon.com/dp/B00SSFWCPA
http://www.amazon.com/dp/1520531230
http://www.amazon.com/dp/B01N4V7SR9
http://www.amazon.com/dp/B00SX58DUI
http://www.amazon.com/dp/B010K7YP62
http://www.amazon.com/dp/B012LAYNNQ
http://www.amazon.com/dp/B00RVX3KY2
http://www.amazon.com/dp/B01MR6SWGW

http://www.amazon.com/dp/B00XF6G4HO
http://www.amazon.com/dp/B01F1472N2
http://www.amazon.com/dp/B00PQ0TUPU
http://www.amazon.com/dp/B00PP8OZJ4
http://www.amazon.com/dp/B00QH7DY4Y
http://www.amazon.com/dp/B01052010G
http://www.amazon.com/dp/B00QDHXN7Q
http://www.amazon.com/dp/B00PO0IQIO

Among others.

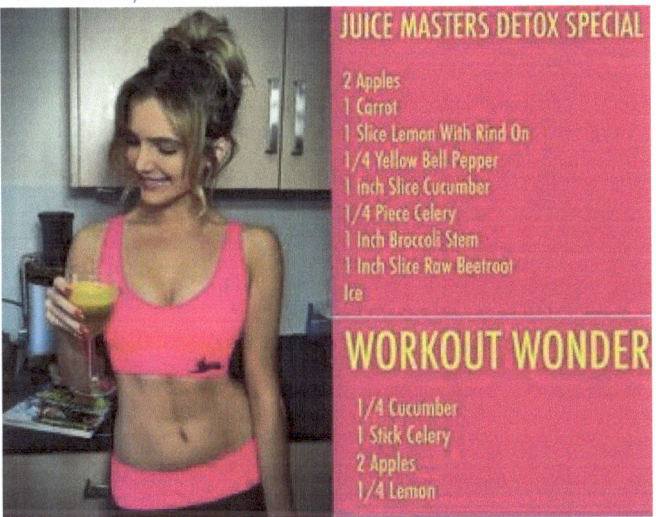

JUICE MASTERS DETOX SPECIAL

2 Apples
1 Carrot
1 Slice Lemon With Rind On
1/4 Yellow Bell Pepper
1 inch Slice Cucumber
1/4 Piece Celery
1 Inch Broccoli Stem
1 Inch Slice Raw Beetroot
Ice

WORKOUT WONDER

1/4 Cucumber
1 Stick Celery
2 Apples
1/4 Lemon

Would you like to know the fastest way to burn fat? Weight loss by healthy and natural means, really comes down to 2 things. By skipping one or both of these things you'll just be wasting your time, if you're looking for the fastest way to burn fat and achieve your weight loss goals. So what are these so-called "secrets" of quick fat loss? Brace yourself. You probably won't like the answer. It comes down to 2 simple things: You have to eat and exercise right! I know it sounds simple but if you have any experience trying to lose weight, you will know that there is a lot more to it than that. Like what sort of exercises burn the fat best? Or, what exactly does "eating right" mean? Good questions, right? The odds are, if you are reading this, you are still looking for answers. You are also one of the 95% of weight loss seekers that have managed to drop a few pounds only to rapidly gain them back. So the lucky 5% have discovered the fastest way to burn fat.

The rest of us are kept in the dark, stuck on a hamster wheel trying diet methods that just don't work! We're led to believe that the answer lies in using quick-fix solutions such as exotic amazon berries, harmful diet pills and prepackaged diet you can get quick results sometimes but they don't last. Once you skip using the pills or stop the diet the weight comes rushing back. I'm not knocking programs like Jenny Craig. I have one slender friend that swears by it. So you don't have to be a TV celebrity to lose weight with that program. But you do have to keep buying and eating those hugely expensive little prepackaged meals. Can you imagine having to do that forever? Because that's what you'll have to do in order to keep the weight off. And forever is an awful long time for most people that's why this fails to be an effective way to lose weight for the long-term. Using a little common sense and going back to the basics will point you in the right direction to finding the fastest way to burn fat.

Most people are looking for a silver bullet when they just need a little education. They need to learn: How to stimulate the body's metabolism so it will burn fat faster. What are negative calories? And which foods require you to burn off calories while you digest them? How certain domestic fruits and vegetables can actually prevent your body from storing fat. The fastest way to burn fat is dependent upon your digestive system working at peak efficiency. And how some whole grains and high-fiber sources can get you there. What exercises are best for quick weight loss and fat burning? And how often do I have to do them? I know of one man that has the answers to all these name is

Oswin Dacosta and he has developed a healthy eating and exercise program that's helped me to lose 37 pounds. I understand your skepticism. I felt the same way, "yet another miracle weight loss system!" right? You're smart to be cautious. There are hundreds of products designed to make you lose money and not weight. But what convinced me to give this a try was that Oswin Dacosta initially created this fat loss system for his own use only. He had no intention of sharing it, but since so many people wanted to know how he managed to lose 50 pounds and stay lean and fit, he decided to go public. So, I liked the idea that he used to be fat, too. He knows what it's like and that's what makes him such a good teacher. Oswin's Fat Burning Furnace isn't just the fastest way to burn fat; it teaches you how to act in the long-term, so that you keep the weight off easily by adopting a simple to maintain and healthy life style. Check out more tips at www.losingbellyfatmisssion.com right away!

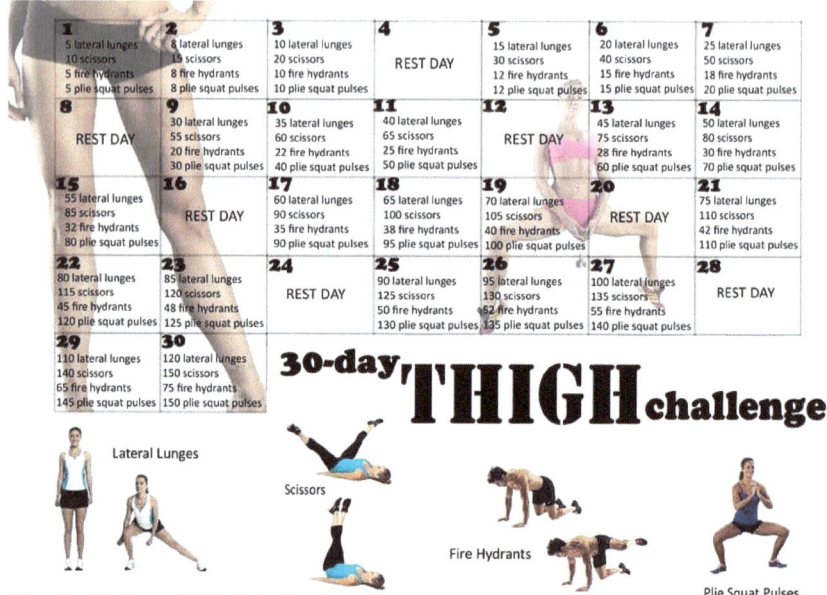

1	2	3	4	5	6	7
5 lateral lunges 10 scissors 5 fire hydrants 5 plie squat pulses	8 lateral lunges 15 scissors 8 fire hydrants 8 plie squat pulses	10 lateral lunges 20 scissors 10 fire hydrants 10 plie squat pulses	REST DAY	15 lateral lunges 30 scissors 12 fire hydrants 12 plie squat pulses	20 lateral lunges 40 scissors 15 fire hydrants 15 plie squat pulses	25 lateral lunges 50 scissors 18 fire hydrants 20 plie squat pulses
8	9	10	11	12	13	14
REST DAY	30 lateral lunges 55 scissors 20 fire hydrants 30 plie squat pulses	35 lateral lunges 60 scissors 22 fire hydrants 40 plie squat pulses	40 lateral lunges 65 scissors 25 fire hydrants 50 plie squat pulses	REST DAY	45 lateral lunges 75 scissors 28 fire hydrants 60 plie squat pulses	50 lateral lunges 80 scissors 30 fire hydrants 70 plie squat pulses
15	16	17	18	19	20	21
55 lateral lunges 85 scissors 32 fire hydrants 80 plie squat pulses	REST DAY	60 lateral lunges 90 scissors 35 fire hydrants 90 plie squat pulses	65 lateral lunges 100 scissors 38 fire hydrants 95 plie squat pulses	70 lateral lunges 105 scissors 40 fire hydrants 100 plie squat pulses	REST DAY	75 lateral lunges 110 scissors 42 fire hydrants 110 plie squat pulses
22	23	24	25	26	27	28
80 lateral lunges 115 scissors 45 fire hydrants 120 plie squat pulses	85 lateral lunges 120 scissors 48 fire hydrants 125 plie squat pulses	REST DAY	90 lateral lunges 125 scissors 50 fire hydrants 130 plie squat pulses	95 lateral lunges 130 scissors 52 fire hydrants 135 plie squat pulses	100 lateral lunges 135 scissors 55 fire hydrants 140 plie squat pulses	REST DAY
29	30					
110 lateral lunges 140 scissors 65 fire hydrants 145 plie squat pulses	120 lateral lunges 150 scissors 75 fire hydrants 150 plie squat pulses					

30-day **THIGH** challenge

Lateral Lunges

Scissors

Fire Hydrants

Plie Squat Pulses

* The number of lateral lunges and fire hydrants indicate the number _per side_
* Modify the above exercises as needed to suit your individual fitness level:
  Add some weights to the lunges and the squat pulses if you like. Break into smaller sets as needed or increase number of repetitions if further challenge is sought.
* The difference between your body this month and next month is what you do over the next 30 days to achieve your goals. Take the challenge.

Do you have a gym membership? Do you go to the gym on a regular basis? If you do, ask yourself this question: "what is my goal?". It seems like a silly question doesn't it? But the truth is that most people who workout do not really have a specific goal in mind. Here is a good goal for you if you need one. Burn fat and build muscle. The only way to change the way your body looks is to have a definite major purpose for working out. When I look around the local gym that I go to, I see people all around me who have been going there for as long as I have who still look the same as they did when I first saw them. It is amazing how quickly you can change the shape of your body when you become focused on how you want to look. It took me about 12 weeks once I figured this out. Your goal when working out should be simple. Burn fat and build muscle. Don't think about looking like a bodybuilder because that is not a realistic goal for the average person. I am simply talking about gaining muscle that changes the shape of your body. For most of my life I wanted to be fit but it all seemed so complicated. Because I had never really gone to the trouble of getting the correct information, I thought it was not possible for me to look fit and athletic.

For years I worked out sporadically but never really changed the way I looked. I was sort of pear-shaped and flabby. I had narrow shoulders and wide hips. It wasn't until I was 32 years old that I literally stumbled onto the right information that changed my thinking about my chances of looking better than I ever thought I could look. Once I began to apply this "new" information, I changed from a flabby, pear-shaped guy, and developed a "V-shaped" body, wider looking shoulders and narrower looking 12 weeks. Listed here are 5 tips that gave me the focus and the determination to accomplish what I had always thought was not possible for me.

1. I got my hands on a training schedule and workout routine (you can find them all over the internet) that I could believe in based on results that others had gotten. Forget about what you hear from other people who think they know all about fitness training and read material from people who have gotten the results that you want.

2. Weight training for about 45 minutes a day for 3 days a week. High intensity, meaning short rest periods between sets and pushing myself to do more weight each week with the same amount of reps.

3. Short 20 minute aerobic workouts 3 alternating days a week. Ideally, first thing in the morning before you eat anything. These must be high intensity, interval type routines, meaning that you must push yourself hard for a minute and then back off for a minute, increasing your intensity (effort) as the routine progresses.

4. Eat 4 to 6 smaller meals each day consisting of a portion of protein and a portion of quality carbohydrates with a couple of good portions of vegetables thrown in. Drink 8 to 10 glasses of water throughout the day and limit your fat intake. Avoid sweets and high fat foods. 5. Take one day off each week and eat whatever you want and don't workout. Rest and enjoy yourself. Of course this is the condensed version and there are a lot more details. But if you are serious about once and for all changing the shape of your body and feeling good about how you look, you will find the details yourself.

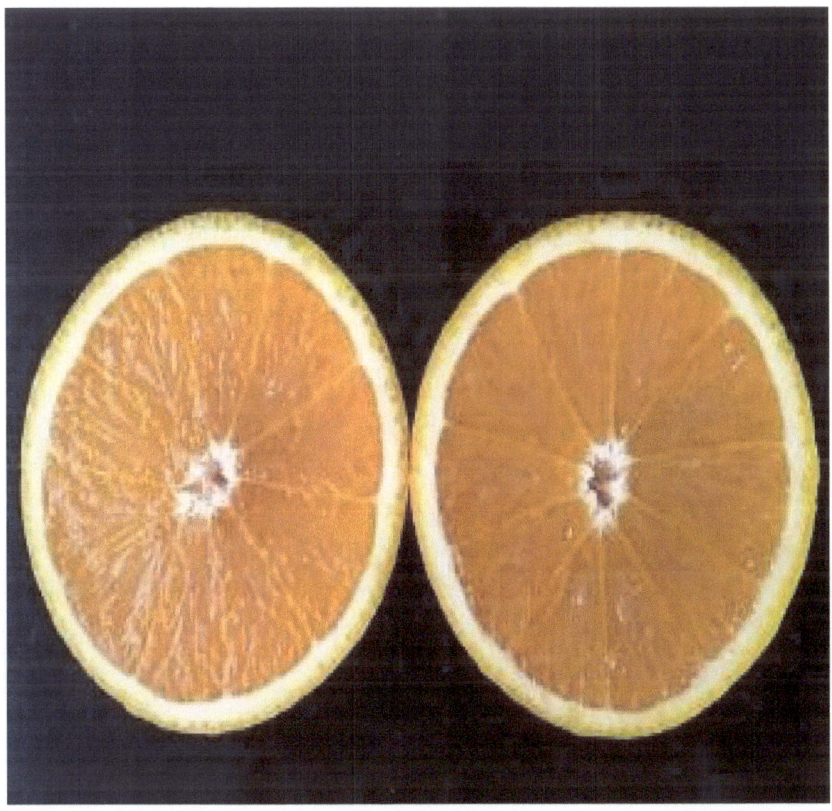

There are many questions that people ask about how to lose fat but at the same time eat well and enjoy life. Despite thoughts to the contrary, this is indeed possible, no matter what you may think right now! However, you do have to use the correct methods and techniques, otherwise your time will just be wasted, and none of us have time to spare these days. Now there are plenty of exercises that you can do to help you lose that fat, whether it is belly fat, or total body fat, but be aware that it probably took you years for your stomach fat to accumulate, and because of this you can know for certain that it is not going to disappear overnight, no matter what you try. We shall concentrate here on fat loss without pills or drugs of any kind, as we believe that this is the best approach for everyone. Now of course, if you are going to start an exercise program or a fat loss diet, then you need to see your medical doctor first to make sure that it is a healthy decision for someone with your particular medical history.

Now, we shall look at the best exercises for losing fat a little later, but first let's just quickly cover what our diet should be for us to lose weight. You probably have a good idea what you should not be eating, and that's junk food. Your body is not made up to live on this kind of food, and it will only lead to serious health problems if you continue to eat junk food. Now, an occasional treat is fine, provided it is just that, occasional! If you know that your will power is a little on the weak side, and having eaten junk food after a long absence you just know you will soon be back on that unhealthy diet, then don't even have the occasional have plenty of food options without fast food. Fruits and vegetables really are good for you, and we have far more choice these days than in the past. We are no longer limited to just the produce grown locally, but because of all the advancements in transport, and the growing of food, we now have a wide selection of vegetables and fruits available for a good portion of the year. By eating a wide selection of fresh produce, you will not get bored with having the same food over and over, so in that way, it has become much easier to become healthy through diet alone.

While meat and dairy products can also be local, unless we live close to farmland, the chances are that our meat products have had further to travel. This is not a problem. However, what is a problem for your diet, is if you eat too much meat, especially the fatty variety like lamb, as animal fat can quite easily increase your cholesterol levels, which is something you do not want to do. So, eat low fat meat, and you probably want to reduce the portion size too. One of the best ways to start losing body fat is to cut down on the amount you eat, and you can do this quite easily. Instead of eating only 3 large meals a day, eat 5 or 6 smaller ones, or 3 smaller meals plus 2 or 3 snacks during the day. You will start to lose weight, provided you are eating less than you normally would. There are some advantages to eating more often during the day.

First of all, you are never more than 2 or 3 hours away from your next intake of food, so even if you get a little peckish, you won't have long to wait for food. Next, these smaller amounts make it easier for your stomach to digest, making it a more efficient process, and giving you energy faster. This will help you to feel more energized, as the energy will be converted from the food faster. Now, you can put this new found energy to good use by exercising, and interval training gives some great results for burning body fat. How does interval training work? Let's imagine you enjoy jogging, and may be you do, then for 5 minutes you would jog along normally, then for the next minute run faster, before returning to the jogging speed for the next 5 minutes, and so on. These bursts of speed will help you to burn off more fat than staying at the same speed all the time, so this is exactly what you want and need.

To lose even more fat, you could do many more fat burning exercises, remembering that a variety is important, not the same exercise all the time. If you choose to do the same exercise every day, you will soon get bored with it, and you may not concentrate enough on the exercise that you are doing, and it may not be as effective for you. Your technique is important, so go back to the basics, and make sure that every exercise is completed as perfectly as possible. Squats are another good way to burn up some of that fat, as squats involve using many different muscles all at the same time. Muscles burn fat when you sue them, so go ahead, use them as often as you can, and your fat level will fall, provided you are not overeating! The stomach vacuum exercise can be done anytime and anywhere, so it is useful to know.

For this you can be stood upright, and you just suck in your stomach as hard as possible, and hold for as long as you can. This gets your stomach muscles back in use, and gets your stomach muscles used to contracting, something which will happen more and more as you lose your belly fat. So, we've mentioned a few exercises that are good for fat loss, and we've discussed the need for a healthy diet. To start with, you need to see your doctor before starting any diet or exercise program, just to make sure, all is well for you, and then there is plenty for you to work on here to lose fat while you eat and live well.

Can You Really Lose Weight in 2 Weeks? Discover the Truth Here & 3 Tips That Can Help You!

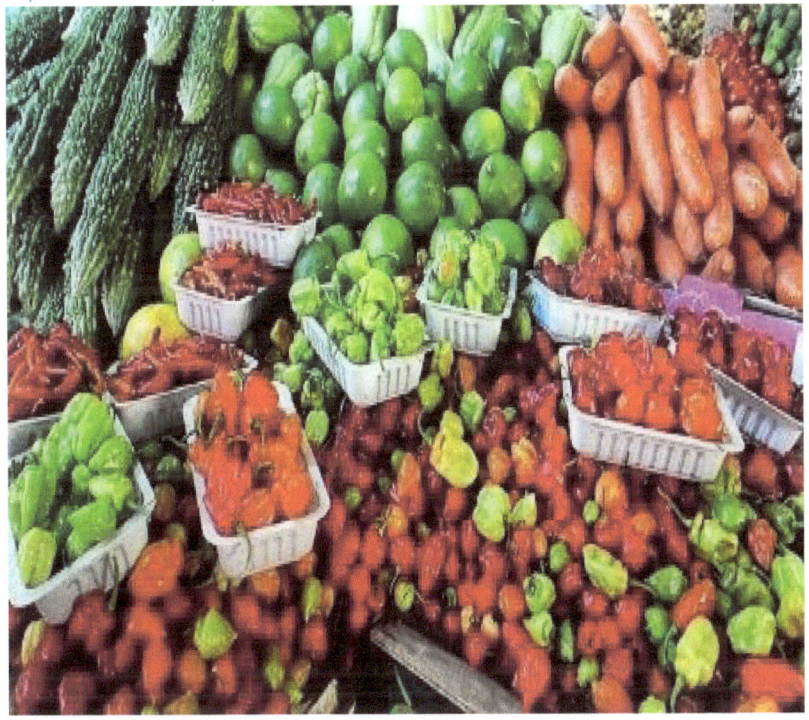

Whilst you can lose weight in 2 weeks, the amount in which you lose will not be a large number. Instead of setting yourself a 2 week goal, you should have a long term goal in place. Anyway, the chances are that if you diet for 2 weeks you will lose a little bit of weight and put it all back on again as soon as you revert back to old habits. A realistic weight loss goal is 1-2 pounds per week, although you will lose more in the first couple of weeks as your body releases water that it was retaining.

In order to ensure you begin losing weight at the quickest rate possible, use these 3 tips in conjunction with an overall weight loss plan.

1. Exercise - Aside from your diet, exercise is the most important component to losing weight successfully. There are hundreds if not thousands of different ways to exercise so you should definitely be able to find something that you enjoy doing. Any time that you burn calories is good for losing weight.

2. Eat More, Not Less - If your plan is to stop eating you will quickly find that your body's metabolism will slow down very quickly and begin holding onto fat. Instead of this, you should look to eat smaller meals more often. Eat as many as 6 meals per day in small portions.

3. Water - Drink plenty of water. It's recommended that you drink 8 glasses of water per day, however, you can drink much more. Water helps speed up your body's metabolism and also helps flush out unwanted toxins. These tips will definitely help you begin losing weight within two weeks and should be used as part of a long term weight management strategy.

Easy Fat Loss For Busy People - 3 Simple Techniques To Burn Fat Fast With A Busy Lifestyle

Crazy work schedule, running a demanding business, having kids, running errands like a crazy person, household duties, and so much more can interfere with anyone who is trying to burn fat, lose weight, and improve their health. Does this describe you? If so, then this article is just for you! Take a couple of quick minutes out of your day and you'll learn in this article 3 simple techniques that helped me (and I'm sure will help you as well) lose pounds of fat regardless of a hectic lifestyle.

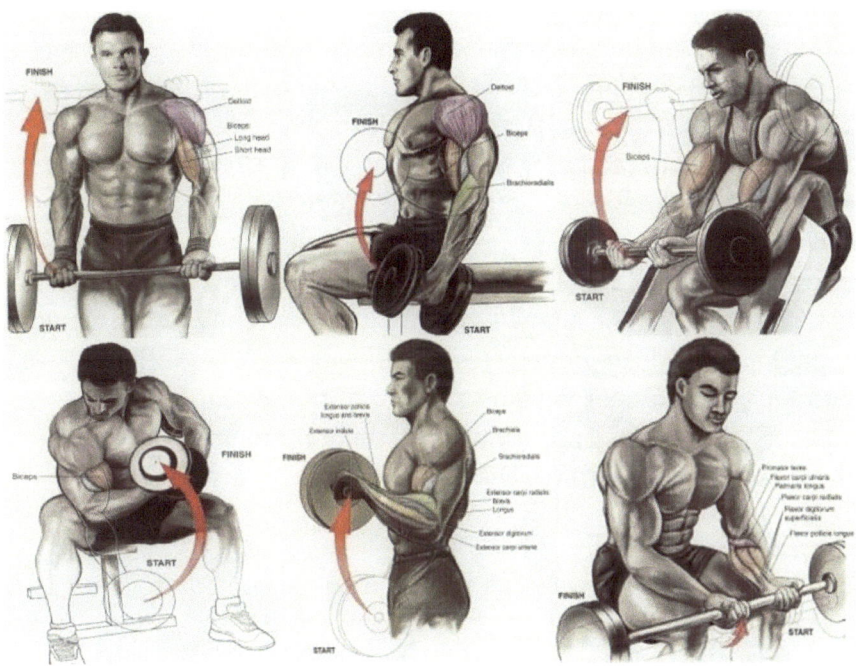

1. The most effective, easiest, and quickest way to exercise... Do body-weight circuit training exercises! These types of exercises are so complete, so convenient, so simple, so affordable, and so everything else it's ridiculous! You can do a quick routine right before you take your shower in the morning prior to starting your day. In fact, these exercise routines mostly are even quicker than taking shower! The reason this type of workout is so powerful and so complete is because you are combining doing both high intensity cardio and resistance training into one. Guess what? It is high intensity cardio and building muscle that will cause pounds of fat to shed off lightning fast. What's even better is that these circuit routines can literally be done in 10-15 minutes... and you'll get a better workout than spending an hour at the gym. Speaking of the gym, that's the other great thing about these exercises: You can do them AT HOME with NO equipment! What I recommend you do with this type of exercise is choose around 3-8 different types of body-weight exercises and do them in a non-stop circuit for 3-5 sets and 30-60 seconds of rest in between. You'll get your heart rate up (cardio), you'll build lean muscle tissue (which means you'll burn fat during the workout AND AFTER the workout is done), and you'll save a ton of time! PLEASE NOTE: Although these exercises are very easy to do and you don't need to use weights in order to do them, I still recommend that you consult your physician first prior to doing them (and especially if you currently have a medical condition). If done improperly (especially with exercises such as squats, push-ups, and burpees to name a few), you can certainly still injure yourself. Also, please ensure you stretch and warm-up prior to doing these exercises, and stretch again after the workout is completed.

2. Take care of 3 birds with one stone... How can you boost your metabolism, ease those strong hunger pangs, and have it all not

interfere with a busy lifestyle? Well, those "3 birds" I just mentioned can all be taken care of by eating smaller meals more frequently! HEY! Stop making that face! I know you've probably heard this tip a billion times before, and you know it, it is so powerful that it deserves to be mentioned the 1,000,000,001 time! The reason you always hear the recommendation of eating more frequently... well... so frequently, is because of those 3 things I mentioned above. Also, when you eat smaller meals, you give your digestive system just enough to properly digest the foods you are eating. If you eat too much at once, this puts a lot of stress on your digestive system... and that will end up causing plenty of problems... including slowing your metabolism down! 3. The right type of diet... What I recommend for you to do is to go on a simple but powerful diet that adjusts to your lifestyle... not the other way around. The best type of diet is one that is based on #2 above, it can instantly be downloaded online, and the only thing you need to get in order to shed pounds of fat fast is NORMAL foods! Also, I recommend a diet that will have you get 100% proper nutrition, without restricting foods, and it should also design a menu plan for you based off of foods YOU like. Why is that important? Well, what better way to lose weight than doing so eating foods you like to eat?

Why Long-Distance Running Won't Burn Fat Fast Enough

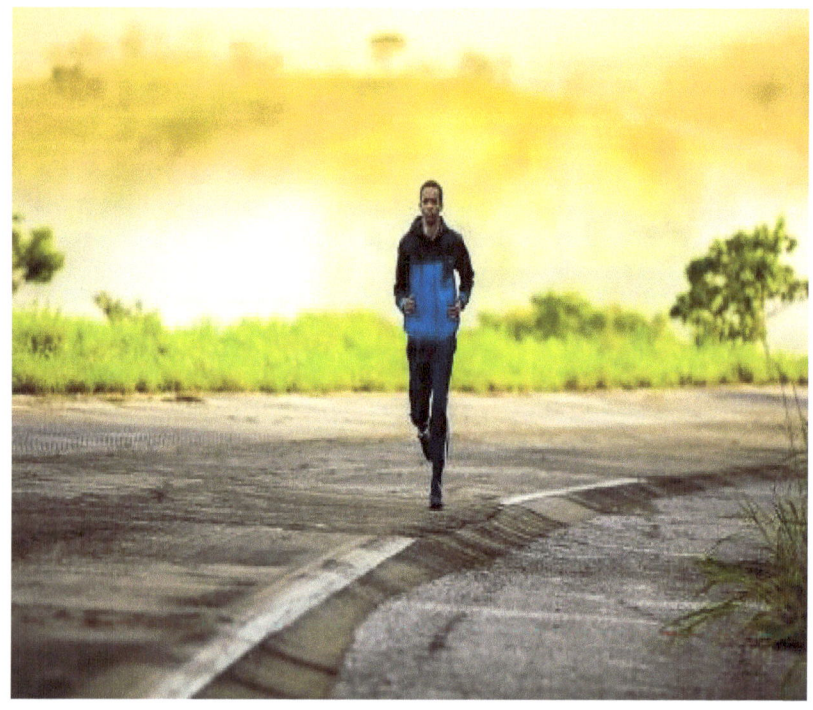

For the longest time, we were under the impression that to lose weight, we need to do several hours of cardiovascular exercises (like long-distance running) a week. After all, cardio burns calories -- strength training is only for bodybuilders. But time, experience, and research are showing that this isn't the case. We now know that long, slow cardiovascular exercises are good for cardiovascular health -- but doesn't really burn fat as quickly as we previously thought. What's worse, limiting yourself to cardiovascular exercises can lead to muscle loss -- and that means shedding weight will become much harder as you get older.

The fact of the matter is that muscle has much more to do with fat burn than we previously thought. After all, muscles are much more metabolically-active than fat, and they burn calories at a regular pace throughout the day, even when you're at rest. This is why it's important to do strength training exercises, such as free weight lifting, as part of your weight loss regimen. What's more, it's best to include interval training exercises in your workout routines, too. Interval training involves exerting maximum effort for short periods of time, followed by short periods of rest or low activity, then exerting maximum effort again. (Hence the name "interval.") It's been proven time and again that a half-hour of interval training burns more calories and builds more muscle than a full hour of cardio. So mix things up and do some strength and interval training as well. And don't forget the other half of the fitness equation -- nutrition -- and take good natural supplements such as Acai berry.

Great Cardio at Home With a Single Exercise!

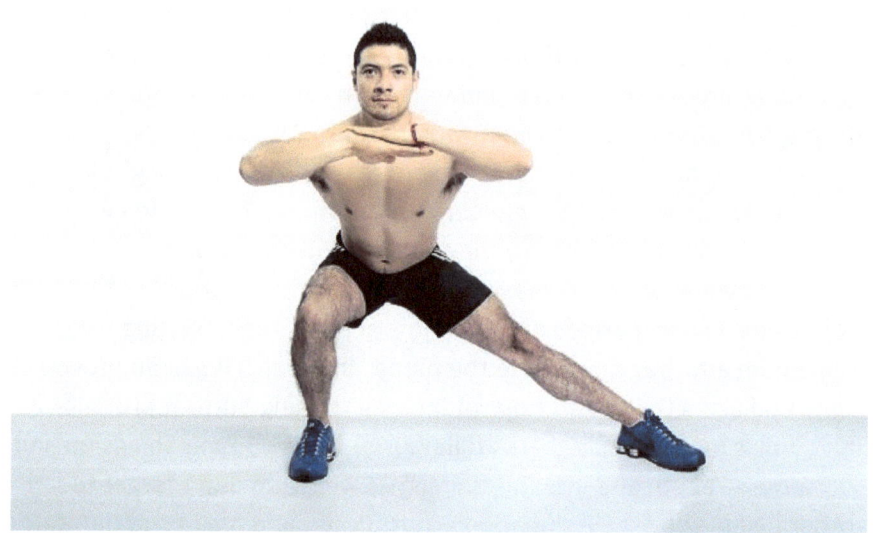

If you think that you have got to go to the trouble to get a $6000 treadmill in order to get a cardio workout then you need to stop reading this article. That kind of thinking is a sign of laziness and spurs excuses as to why you should not workout. Forget about equipment because all you need is your living room floor or back yard and the availability of yourself to get a hard hitting cardio workout! Read on if I have your attention. The Squat Thrust If you are wanting a cardio exercise to do at home then you have found it with this drill my friend. The squat thrust is a body weight exercise that is sure to get you breathing hard in a hurry. This particular exercise is a calisthenic that thoroughly challenges your muscular system while getting your level of perceived exertion up very fast at the same time.

To perform the squat thrust you will want to stand with your feet at about a shoulder width distance apart in length. From here simply crouch down to place your hands on the ground in front of you. From here simply kick your feet back behind you bringing yourself into an upright push up position. Next, simply kick your feet back up to crouch your body again to stand up. All 3 of these steps equate to a single repetition with this total body blasting cardio strength drill. After performing this drill for a good 15 to 20 reps you will see just what I mean when I say "cardio." Take the time to include this exercise in your arsenal of in home conditioning workouts. If you are serious about results then you have got to train like you are serious about getting them.

Squat thrusts are great for getting you into tip top physical condition for you to be ready for most any physical task you decide to take on. If you haven't already begun to use squat thrusts and other great body weight exercises for your cardio workouts at home then you could be missing out and potentially losing a boat load of money on unnecessary equipment that is going to give you nothing more than an added dust collection. Take the time to learn more on this subject by accessing the rest of my articles on the issue for free. Remember that most anyone can train hard, but only the best train smart my friend!

These are some of my other books below, and my website is
www.LosingBellyFatMission.com :

https://www.amazon.com/dp/B06XB4WHZX
http://www.amazon.com/dp/B06X9LXBB8
http://www.amazon.com/dp/B06WLK7497
http://www.amazon.com/dp/B06W54JKQN
http://www.amazon.com/dp/B06X6DJ9K3
http://www.amazon.com/dp/B06WGNJ9N3
http://www.amazon.com/dp/B06W549TBD
http://www.amazon.com/dp/B06VTF5DQJ
http://www.amazon.com/dp/B06WRPSBKK
http://www.amazon.com/dp/B06WD194JR
http://www.amazon.com/dp/B06WCZTK7Y
http://www.amazon.com/dp/B06X3QN1HT
http://www.amazon.com/dp/B01N19WBF2
http://www.amazon.com/dp/B01N2AVECA
http://www.amazon.com/dp/B01N4VZIAV
http://www.amazon.com/dp/B00QJJFS1C
http://www.amazon.com/dp/B01EMNO2MW
http://www.amazon.com/dp/B00SSFWCPA
http://www.amazon.com/dp/1520531230
http://www.amazon.com/dp/B01N4V7SR9
http://www.amazon.com/dp/B00SX58DUI
http://www.amazon.com/dp/B010K7YP62
http://www.amazon.com/dp/B012LAYNNQ
http://www.amazon.com/dp/B00RVX3KY2
http://www.amazon.com/dp/B01MR6SWGW
http://www.amazon.com/dp/B00XF6G4HO
http://www.amazon.com/dp/B01F1472N2

http://www.amazon.com/dp/B00PQ0TUPU
http://www.amazon.com/dp/B00PP8OZJ4
http://www.amazon.com/dp/B00QH7DY4Y
http://www.amazon.com/dp/B01052010G
http://www.amazon.com/dp/B00QDHXN7Q
http://www.amazon.com/dp/B00PO0IQIO

Among others.

www.ingramcontent.com/pod-product-compliance
Lightning Source LLC
Chambersburg PA
CBHW050931290526
45792CB00002B/972

* 9 7 8 1 5 4 4 2 6 8 1 6 3 *